THIS TIME, DON'T FIGHT

This Time, Don't Fight

Dana-Susan Crews

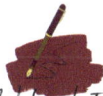

Ashland Ink

Published by Ashland Ink Publishing
209 West 2nd Street #177
Fort Worth TX 76102
www.ashlandink.com

Published in the United States of America

ISBN: 978-1-963514-14-8

Dedication

This book is dedicated to my children, Morgan and Dylan, and my whole family, who didn't let us struggle alone. It is also dedicated to our friends who are like family to us and the medical team at Texas Health Harris Methodist Hospital in downtown Fort Worth.

A special and incredible thank you to Miranda, Karen, the Thomison Family, and our neighbors in Marine Creek Ranch in north Fort Worth for saving a life. You are my heroes.

Dana-Sue

Introduction

You will not have to fight this battle (2 Chronicles 20:17)

In 2003, our family began a fight against an enemy too big for us. We all fought together, along with Jesus, to conquer stage four cancer when it struck. There is a time to fight. There is a time to pick up a sword and march out onto a battlefield and, with as much determination as you can, wage war on the evil around you.

But there is also a time to let God do the fighting, to let everything go and get out of the way while He conquers your enemy for you.

This story is about a sudden battle against a fierce destroyer, and all the same characters were once again involved. This time, we were older and very tired. This time, although we turned to our faith again, we laid down our swords and let the Captain of the Army of the Lord fight.

Heart of Gold

On Sunday, March 2, 2025, our world changed and it will never be the same again.

Before this happened, Bill and I were in Washington, D.C., lobbying on Capitol Hill with more than 300 pediatric cancer advocates through the Alliance for Childhood Cancer. Many decades ago, Bill was seven years old when his five-year-old sister was diagnosed with leukemia. One year later, Michelle took her final breath at the age of six.

When I first met Bill, I thought I was lucky to finally meet someone who understood the impact of childhood cancer. We were both seven years old when we had a younger sibling diagnosed. He and I knew what it was like to be afraid, to be confused, to be devastated by great sickness. But I was the lucky one because my baby brother survived.

One day, I asked Bill to share some of his memories of his sister. It was so sweet to hear him talk about her upbeat personality, her love of animals, and her feisty courage. He talked about swimming with her, playing board games together, and chasing chickens on their grandparents' ranch. Of all the memories he shared, though, the most vivid of all was that of an eight-year-old boy bending down to a coffin to kiss his sister's cold cheek.

Her death changed everything. It crushed the life out of his parents. They managed to go on, though. After all, they had two sons who needed them to be good parents. But losing a child is the most horrifying experience a parent can endure. Of course, they would never be the same again. And neither would Bill. There was a hole in his heart that could never be filled again.

Because both of us had been introduced to childhood cancer as kids, and because we had gotten married, we believed God put us together for a reason. Maybe part of that reason was to get involved somehow in fundraising or advocacy for pediatric cancer.

Before I met Bill, I did some projects for childhood cancer patients and hosted some fun gift basket drives for area hospitals. I especially enjoyed getting my young students involved in these projects. I truly believe that a heart for philanthropy starts at a young age, and my hope was to show my students that they had the power to make a difference in the world.

Around 2002, Bill and I began talking about starting a small publishing company to publish children's books written by children with cancer. Not long after we started working on our business proposal, one of Bill's college friends died of leukemia. Only a few months later, Bill was diagnosed with stage four non-Hodgkin lymphoma. We learned a lot during that time of war about the AYA (adolescent/young adult) cancer community and the challenges of facing a life-threatening illness as a young adult. This only solidified our desire to do some good for kids with cancer.

Bill's cancer journey gave us the opportunity to volunteer with the Leukemia & Lymphoma Society and MD Anderson Cancer Center. We worked to raise awareness and funding with a heavy emphasis on childhood and AYA cancers.

Finally, at the end of 2020, we remembered our original dream of starting a publishing company for kids with cancer, and with the lockdowns of COVID, I realized I had the time to do the work. Bell Asteri Publishing was born, and over the next few years, we saw it grow quickly and flourish in ways we could not have imagined when we first thought it up two decades before.

We also got more involved in advocacy. Previously, we had done some advocacy at the state and local levels, but mostly for blood cancers. Now, we were taking a deep dive into advocacy for every childhood cancer. We both joined the National Advisory Council for Gold Together for Childhood Cancer at the American Cancer Society, and we became active members of the Coalition Against Childhood Cancer. Our lobbying moved from just the state level to the national level.

At the end of February 2025, we made another trip to Washington, D.C. with the Alliance for Childhood Cancer. The Alliance brings together advocacy organizations, medical and scientific organizations, and groups working collaboratively to advance research and policies to improve outcomes for children and teens with cancer.

For Bill and me, this trip was special because not only did we get to lobby for this very important nonpartisan cause, but we also got to visit with some of our favorite people. We have discovered that the Gold Together group and the many others we have met over the years through our work have become a family to us. We see them in September in D.C., also, but we have monthly meetings thanks to Zoom.

The February trip was filled with both fun times and work. On Friday, February 28, we joined fellow Texans to speak to the offices of Ted Cruz, John Cornyn, and to several members of the House of Representatives about some important legislation. When I think about it now, it is hard to believe that Bill was able to walk all over Washington, D.C. He was able to fly there and back. He was himself. Nothing seemed strange at all.

On Saturday, March 1, we slowly got out of bed and walked a fairly long distance to have brunch. Then we walked back to our hotel with no trouble at all. We got to the airport and snacked on some chips and guacamole. We got on our flight home and had a smooth and easy trip back to DFW airport.

When we got home at about 9:30 p.m., I remember thinking how glad I was that I married someone who has a heart of gold, who loves the childhood cancer community as much as I do, and who always gives generously and cheerfully.

That night, I thought about how glad I was to be home and sleep in my own bed and how I was hopeful not to wake up early the next day. Bill, on the other hand, had agreed to go on a six-mile run with our daughter Morgan. He hadn't run in a few days, so he was happy to go out and do what he loves.

It is hard to imagine that Saturday night now. I had no idea what was around the corner, that Death was lurking and about to pounce.

Don't Leave Me

Marriage is not easy. Two people with their own ideas and differences come together and they vow to stay together through the good times and bad, through the rich times and poor times, through the sick times and healthy times - til death parts them.

On June 1, 1996, I vowed to love Bill in sickness and in health, and at the time, I had no idea that he was standing before me with cancer growing in his body. We wouldn't know for years until his lymphoma decided to get out of control and attack his entire body.

In 2003, when we discovered that he was full of cancer, our family fought. All of us fought hard. My kids were only five and three years old, and they had to learn how to be tough soldiers. They had to learn about sickness and dying way too early in life. But I guess Bill and I did too. Through my kids, I learned that being a little kid with a parent with cancer is really difficult. I had already known that being a childhood cancer sibling was rough, but seeing what my kids endured, I discovered the wretchedness of cancer in other ways. Cancer is just plain evil.

We wrote a book about our fight. And that is exactly what it was. It was a huge fight. It was a war filled with many long and difficult battles. Sometimes in life, you just have to fight.

During that time, I learned how to love my husband in sickness. I already knew how to love him in health. He had been an athlete his entire life. We had volunteered coaching a local swim team when we first got married, and we also competed ourselves at the master's level. Loving him in health was a great thrill. Loving him in sickness was the most profound kind of love I ever knew.

I was only 33 years old, but much of the time during his cancer battles, I felt so much older and worn out. Our story had a pretty incredible ending, though. Bill didn't stay down. He beat lymphoma. He became an Ironman triathlete. So did I. Once again, I loved him in health. We knew the extremes of both sickness and health. Stage four incurable cancer is extreme. Ironman is extreme. That was who we were - extreme. It was the "go big or go home" mantra, and we lived it every single day.

In 2018, we became empty nesters. The day after our youngest, Dylan, graduated from The Woodlands High School, we moved to Fort Worth. Our neighborhood has some decent running trails, and we have a small lake with a paved running trail that goes all around the lake. Bill and I don't typically run together because his schedule has been challenging with work. For years, he would rise at 4:00 in the morning and spend some time drinking coffee and doing a Bible devotion, and then head out on a run. He really enjoyed those early morning runs in the dark. They gave him the chance to be alone and have a bit of an escape from the pressures of life before heading to the office.

On the weekends, though, he would often run with our daughter Morgan. They enjoyed training together for foot races.

She had been living in McKinney, which is about an hour away from Fort Worth. But in February of 2025, she accepted a position in downtown Fort Worth. On Sunday, February 23, she and Bill ran the Cowtown half marathon together. I was in the Sundance Square area with my friend Harris and his kids cheering on runners. His wife, Melissa, was also running, and we had decided to go out and cheer on our people.

Nothing was unusual about that day or that race. Morgan had a goal of finishing in under two hours, and when I saw her, I was excited because she was making her time, but I was also a bit confused because Bill wasn't with her. About a minute later, he ran by, and I asked if he was ok. He smiled and said he was fine but that he had just gotten a bit winded. They both had a great finish time and finished in much less than two hours.

A few days after the race, we flew to D.C., and everything there seemed normal. Bill was himself. Nothing seemed wrong at all. I almost get shaky when I think back to those moments. Lying beneath the surface was a monster. This time it wasn't cancer, but it was just as scary. Maybe even scarier.

Exactly one week after the Cowtown half marathon, Morgan and Bill set out to run an easy six miles. She had texted the day before, as we were boarding our flight, and asked if Bill wanted to run with her the next day. He was very tired, but he also really wanted to run since he hadn't run in a few days, so he agreed to go.

On Saturday night, after we returned home and unpacked, Bill headed to bed. It was 10:00, and we were both exhausted, but I wanted to unwind by watching a show for a bit. I was a little nauseated, and before I went into the living room, I lay my head on Bill's lap and he held me for a minute.

It's so strange to remember that moment now. Strange because as he held me, I thought about how nice it felt to just have a little hug for a minute, and how I wanted to spend more time doing that and less time being so busy. I told him goodnight, and then I went to watch a show for 20 minutes before going to bed.

Sunday morning arrived, and it was one of those super windy Fort Worth days. I was glad I wasn't going running that morning. I got up, and Bill was sitting on the couch, drinking coffee. Because he was running with Morgan, he didn't go out super early. They had decided to go a bit later in the morning. I grabbed coffee and returned to my bed to just relax. A little later, Bill came in and changed into running clothes. I don't remember if I even spoke to him. Did I say, "Have a nice run," or "See you later," or anything at all? I heard the front door open and close, and I knew that he and Morgan were running.

Right after they left, I decided to get up and start taking down all the Valentine's Day decor in the house. It was March 2, and it was time to put up some Easter decorations. Some of the outdoor decorations needed to come in, so I made a last-minute decision to get dressed. While I put out Easter decor, I thought it might be nice to have another cup of coffee and sit on the porch. My phone was silenced, but I kept getting buzzed on my watch. I didn't realize those buzzes were phone calls. I get buzzed when our Ring app sounds, and since I'd been going in and out of the front door, I figured that was why my watch was buzzing. I could not have been more wrong.

Moments later, someone was ringing my doorbell and then banging on the door. I knew something was terribly wrong. I opened the door, and there stood a woman I had never met speaking words I will never forget. "Your husband had a heart attack. Your daughter is there with him. She has been trying to call you for several minutes."

In an instant, I felt a panic hit me like I never had before. "What? Where are they? Where is my phone?" I grabbed my phone and noticed about 20 missed calls, and then ran out the door with this woman and jumped into her car. On the way, she told me that she was a nurse and that she had been driving by and had seen Bill on the ground, and she pulled over to begin CPR. His heart was not beating, and he was not breathing on his own.

The many missed calls on my phone were from numbers I didn't know. I had many voicemails, but I didn't listen. Instead, I called my mom. "Bill had a heart attack, and his heart stopped beating. I need you to come to Fort Worth, Mom. Bill is dying!"

Just 1.4 miles down the road from my house, we arrived on the scene. Karen pulled up onto the street, and I jumped out. There were police officers, firefighters, and paramedics everywhere. They surrounded Bill, who was on the ground, covered in blood. Morgan was standing with several neighbors I don't know, and she was crying. I hugged her. I tried to run to Bill, but a paramedic stopped me. Then I fell to the ground and began begging Jesus to save my husband's life.

A woman who was also a nurse sat on the ground with me. She had also been administering CPR to Bill. She and the nurse who picked me up were just passersby and had just happened to drive by when he collapsed. They had been taking turns doing CPR to try to keep oxygen going to his brain before the ambulance arrived. Later, I would learn that her name was Miranda. She started praying with me. In fact, the people standing with Morgan were also praying. But while we were praying, Bill was on the ground in a pool of his blood, and he was dead.

One of the paramedics approached me. I can't remember what he said or asked me. He began telling me they were taking him to a hospital downtown. "We are going to Harris," he said. I had no idea where that was. But Miranda did, and she listened closely to everything being said. And she told the paramedic she would ensure that Morgan and I got there.

Moments later, the paramedic said they were putting Bill into the ambulance and that he would let me get on and tell him goodbye quickly before they took off. "Quickly!" He made sure I understood I had to move fast. I got on, and Bill was hooked up to all kinds of equipment. He had blood all over his face and head. One of the paramedics was working on him, and I asked her if he could hear me. She told me she didn't know, but that I should just talk to him and fast because they had to go. I found a spot to kiss his face, and then I whispered in his ear, "Fight, Memo, fight."

Memo. My Memo. That's one of my nicknames for him. It's how you say "Bill" in Spanish. Fight. That's what I needed him to do. We have fought for his life before. This was so much more urgent and way more frightening, especially because moments before, he was literally dead. Sudden cardiac death.

I got out of the ambulance. I handed my phone to Morgan and told her to call our neighbor Kevin to see if he could drive us to the hospital. No one there that day believed Morgan and I should be driving. Miranda offered to take us, but I thought that it might be best to ride with Kevin or at least let our neighbors on our street know what was happening.

Everything was so overwhelming. I could hardly believe this was real and not some crazy dream. The ambulance was screaming down the road to take my dying husband away, to fight for his life, which had already been taken from him minutes before. I saw one of the first responders spraying something on the path and sweeping up his blood. His blood. Once upon a time, there was cancer in his blood. Now, his blood was on the sidewalk, and his heart had stopped beating.

"Don't leave me, Memo."

Tell Your Heart to Beat

Kevin and Sheila are our neighbors across the street. They were waiting for us in our driveway when Miranda dropped us off. I ran inside the house to grab my wallet. Suddenly, I was thinking about the logistics of everything. I would need an insurance card and money. While I was grabbing my wallet, Miranda told Kevin where to take us.

I quickly grabbed my wallet and ran back outside to jump into Kevin's truck and sit next to Morgan. She was wearing her running clothes. She was shaking. As we drove away, she got on the phone to call Dylan. It was torture to think about my son getting that call. He was preparing to head to New Mexico to fly a T6 for the Navy. He's a naval aviator in Corpus Christi and had been excited about this next phase in his career. I struggled to concentrate on what Morgan was saying to him, and then she handed me the phone.

"Dib," I said, using my nickname for him, "I'm sorry. Can you get to Fort Worth?" He told me he was texting his commanding officer and getting on the next flight to DFW.

I cannot imagine what Kevin and Sheila were thinking during

all of this. I began chattering about how ironic it was that Bill had just told me that if he ever died, I should hope he died on an oil rig so I would get way more insurance money. Then I made the comment that I would rather pay millions of dollars to keep him. I couldn't stop begging God to let him live.

Morgan was crying and beginning to say that the entire incident was her fault because she had complained about the wind and asked Bill to stop for a moment.

And you see, her perspective of the story was traumatic. She and her dad had started their run with no issues, but the wind was picking up. Fort Worth wind can be fierce, and when you are running slightly uphill with it in your face, it is awful. She began to complain about how difficult it was to run in the wind and then asked if they could stop for a second. That's when Bill said, "I'm dizzy." Then, as most people having a heart attack do, he made some strange movements, almost like a seizure, and then collapsed on the ground. He fell backward and slammed the back of his head into the concrete sidewalk. Morgan ran to him, screaming. He was unresponsive. He had fallen on top of his phone, and she hadn't brought her phone with her, so she was there alone with no help and no way to call for help. Her dad was bleeding and not breathing.

Suddenly, a young family on their way to church drove by, and Morgan flagged them down. They pulled over and called 911. Miracles happen more often than we realize. Was it luck or a miracle that not long after this family stopped, two other neighbors drove by, and they both happened to be registered nurses? Karen was the first to stop, and she began CPR. Then Miranda drove by, and she and Karen took turns doing CPR. They did not get a pulse, but their quick and quality CPR delivered oxygen to his brain. It is impossible to know how long he was without oxygen to the brain, but had they not arrived when they did, he would not have survived.

As a mom, the thought of my daughter being there all alone, covered in her dad's blood, sweat, and a tiny tear that rolled down his cheek, tortures my soul. She had used these good Samaritans' phones to call me over and over again, but I had not answered my phone. Her dad died in front of her, and she was surrounded by strangers. Yet these strangers were sent from God. They all prayed with her and for her dad while her mom was not there.

Although it seemed like Kevin was driving way faster than the speed limit to get us to the hospital, it also felt like it took a hundred years. My brother Luke called. I had thought he and his wife, Virginia, were in Brazil, but I was off by one week. They were still in town, and he had gone out looking for Bill when my mom called him. I told him to meet us at the hospital.

Kevin pulled up to the entrance to the emergency room. Morgan and I jumped out and ran in. The doors opened to a security guard. I didn't even get out my name or Bill's full name. "My husband was brought in," I said as I handed them my phone and wallet to be scanned. They told me that a chaplain was going to meet me through the doors to the left.

Morgan and I walked through the doors to the left, and there was a chaplain named Stephanie. She was very calm and kind. She escorted us to a small room, and I asked if Bill was alive. She didn't answer. She simply told me that someone would come out to talk to Morgan and me soon. She had us sit on a sofa in the tiny room, and she brought us a cup of water. I asked her to bring Morgan a warm blanket because Morgan was shivering.

My daughter and I sat next to each other, feeling extreme fear and pain. I desperately wanted to take away the trauma she'd just experienced. She had witnessed her dad die on the spot. She was shaking, partly from the cold and partly from the trauma. I begged her to sip some water. I told her I would find her some hot tea. But all she could do was burst into tears and cry out that all of this was her fault.

"I complained about the wind, Mom," she cried. I did my best to help her think logically. If complaining about the wind could cause sudden cardiac death, he would have died long ago, because I also complain about the wind when we run together. But then she cried all the more, saying that the last words her dad ever heard her speak were complaints. The truth is, we should all remind ourselves that we don't know how long we have with the people we love, and we should be kind way more often. But her complaints about the wind were not mean. They were justified.

My brother Luke walked in. He sat next to Morgan on the tiny sofa. I was on a chair next to them, holding Morgan's hand and trying to be calm, but on the inside, I was screaming in agony. Luke was comforting for both of us. I was glad that someone who could listen to everything we would be hearing from the physicians was there with us.

Soon, a nurse came to get us, and we all three walked back to the room where Bill was hooked up to all kinds of machines. By now, he needed the machines to breathe for him, to pump blood for him, to beat his broken heart that refused to beat on its own. Even his kidneys were dead. But the most critical issue now was his brain. How long did his brain go without oxygen? Was there any hope at all, or were we facing a decision about donating his organs?

I have lost count of how many doctors and nurses were in and out of the room, and how many times I answered the questions asked repeatedly. *Does he smoke? Does he do any drugs or take any medications? Does he drink alcohol, and how much?* Every single person who asked me this was given the exact same answers, and I was sick of telling them the same things. *No, he doesn't smoke. He takes a multivitamin every morning. He will occasionally have a beer, but no, he's not a heavy drinker.*

When I think about how this must have looked, I'm sure everyone on the medical team couldn't believe that they were dealing with a man with a healthy diet, a marathoner, and an Ironman triathlete. They usually see older patients, overweight patients, young people who do heavy amounts of drugs, and folks who eat awful diets and live sedentary lifestyles.

But over and over, I let them all know one truth about him that I'm sure was not a common answer there. From 2003-2004, he had stage four lymphoma that had metastasized to his bones, and part of his treatment plan that lasted for almost three years included eight rounds of intensive chemotherapy. One of the chemotherapy agents was extremely toxic and had the potential to cause heart failure. Bill had received a lifetime limit of it in only six months. Although more than twenty years had gone by, there was a high probability that the effects of chemo had finally caught up to him.

A nurse named Debby was there with Bill the entire time. No matter who else walked in, Debby stayed. She was a runner. She attempted to get me and then Morgan to talk about running and running clubs in the area. She was energetic, and I thought how she would be a fun person to hang out with if we weren't in this situation.

Morgan's friend arrived to help support her. He was very calm, and I was glad he was there because I had to concentrate on Bill and couldn't be there for Morgan. She was not emotionally able to stay in that room with her dad in that condition for too long. She would come in briefly and then walk out. Having her friend there meant that Luke and I could stay with Bill and be sure to listen closely to everything they said.

A cardiologist named Dr. Amin came to talk to us. He had a soft, tranquil demeanor. He told us this was a critical situation and that brain function was a pressing concern. Bill's brain had been without oxygen for a few minutes and maybe up to 12 minutes. If that were the case, this was the end. But because he had received high-quality CPR quickly, it was likely that oxygen had been restored within less than five minutes after his sudden death. The paramedics had shocked him three times when they arrived. He should not even be alive at all. Only one percent of people who experience a heart attack with cardiac death outside of a hospital survive. It wasn't a big one, but there was still a fighting chance.

Dr. Amin told us that they would be taking Bill to the cath lab soon. Then, another physician walked in with a team, and they began sewing Bill's head. When he fell, he suffered a five-centimeter gash on the back of his head.

"Can he feel that?" I asked. Nurse Debby said that he probably could feel it, but that this was the least of my worries. Every chance I had, I walked over to Bill to hold his hand and tell him that we were in the room and that I needed him to keep fighting. "Tell your heart to beat, Memo."

Wake Up!

During the time in the emergency room, I suddenly realized that I would need to contact Bill's boss to let him know that, obviously, Bill would not be at work the next day.

I had Bill's phone, but I couldn't remember his password. He changes his password often, and none of the old ones I remembered worked. So, without being able to hack into his phone, I had no way of finding his boss' contact information. I tried logging onto LinkedIn to find him there and message him, but my app wasn't working. I tried looking online at his company website, but no contact information was there either. I began to panic. Nurse Debby turned to me and said, "This is not urgent. What is happening is that you are trying to find something you can do in a helpless situation, so you are concentrating on contacting his employer. Don't worry about that right now."

Although I knew she was right, I had to do something, and if that was the only thing I could claim control over at the moment, I would find that phone number and call his boss. I remembered that my friends in The Woodlands knew his boss,

Jim. I called Ann and told her what had happened and asked if she could find Jim's phone number. She said she would ask her husband and text me. In a few minutes, I got her text and called Jim. Thankfully, he answered the call, and I told him what was happening with Bill. I don't know why it made me feel so relieved to get that task done, but it did.

At some point, someone from the administration came to get our insurance information and get me to sign several papers. I didn't even pay attention to what I was signing. I knew it was all legal stuff about privacy and payments. I also gave her my contact information and Morgan and Dylan's and told her that any of us was permitted to get information about Bill.

Finally, the medical team came to wheel Bill out of the room and to the cath lab. We were escorted to a private waiting room. Morgan's friend bought us all lunch and had it in the room, and I was glad that Morgan agreed to eat something. My mom arrived. As soon as she walked in, I hugged her and started crying. I hated that she had to drive all the way from Huntsville by herself, but I knew that if I was about to become a widow, I could not do this without her support.

My sister-in-law, Virginia, had gone to the airport to pick up Dylan, and as they approached the hospital parking garage, they called Luke, and he said he would head down to escort them to our waiting room. Morgan had stepped out for a few minutes, too. With just my mom and me in the room, one of the doctors came in to tell us that they could not put in a stent. He said that at least three of the main arteries to Bill's heart were blocked. He said he would need bypass surgery.

Morgan returned, and then another doctor walked in. He explained a bit more about Bill's condition, and then he stopped and looked at Morgan and told her that she helped to save her dad's life that day. He told her that if she hadn't been with him, that if he had been alone, he would be dead. Her quick reaction to flag down neighbors saved his life. I really wanted to hug that doctor for saying this to my broken daughter. I thanked him and he left.

Luke walked in with Dylan and Virginia. I hugged them, and then Dylan sat next to me. I wanted to grab both of my kids and hold them so bad. I hated that they were having to endure this. I told everyone what the doctors had said. I realized as I spoke that we might soon be planning a funeral, but I also had incredible hope that he would survive. But that was not enough for me.

I didn't want Bill to survive and not have a great quality of life. I wanted him to survive and be himself. I wanted to know that his brain was working right, and in fact, that was a major problem for the team. His brain function had to be tested to determine if he could even have the bypass surgery. So, Bill was being sent to the cardiovascular ICU, where he would remain paralyzed and sedated, hooked up to a ventilator until brain function could be determined.

Soon, everyone left except for my mom, my children, and me. The four of us were not strangers to being together, fighting for Bill's life. More than two decades before, we fought. Here we were again, doing our best to find the strength to bravely endure.

A nurse came to tell us that we could visit Bill in the ICU, two at a time. She told us he was not conscious but that we could talk to him. I let Morgan and Dylan go first, and then my mom and I went in. He was so white and cold. He looked like death, but when I kissed his cheek, I felt him in there. I begged him to live. I begged him to wake up.

Nights in the ICU

Death is certain, just like taxes. Most of us don't walk around thinking about either, but every April 15, we are forced to remember to pay taxes, and sometimes, we are forced to realize our immortality.

When the sun no longer shone through the big window in Bill's room in the cardiovascular intensive care unit, the darkness became a bit bolder. On that first night, the man next to him coded. Everyone on staff ran in to save his life.

But throughout that two-week stay, I would hear two others die and many "code blue" alerts. The medical staff at this hospital was made up of some incredibly intelligent people. I wondered how these nurses managed to forget their jobs when they went home. How did they escape the pressure and pain of working in the ICU with the sights and sounds of death and dying every day?

On that first night, I had decided to stay at the hospital. I did not want to leave Bill there alone. What if he woke up and was scared? Or what if he took his final breath and no one was there with him in his final moments?

Of course, this was not the first time I'd been in this situation. More than 20 years before, I had been torn between two worlds. At home were my children, who needed their mom but were at least being cared for by their grandma. At the hospital was Bill, maybe dying of cancer. I did not want him to die alone. Here I was again. My children were adults now, and they were with their grandma at my house. I wanted to be with them, but I decided to be with Bill. There would be no way he would ever be alone. He needed us.

After we all had a brief visit with Bill, we went home. I grabbed a few items to place in an overnight bag. Dylan was in charge of going out to get everyone dinner. Morgan was in charge of going to pick up my dog, Bella. I asked Kevin and Sheila to take me back to the hospital because I'm not able to drive well at night. I hated leaving them all. I was exhausted, and I just wanted to hold my dog and sleep in my bed.

I arrived at the ICU. A nurse was in the room with Bill, changing out some of the 10 bags of medications on his IV pole. There was a "recliner" by the window with a pile of white blankets that had been on Bill in the emergency room. I put my bag down on the floor, and then I picked up the blankets, sat on the chair, and held the blankets in my arms. I was hoping they smelled like him. A pillow was on the windowsill. It had drops of his blood on it.

When the nurse walked out, I got up and stood beside Bill, holding his hand. By now, I was wearing his wedding band on my right hand. It didn't fit, but I kept it on my index finger. At home, Dylan was wearing Bill's James Avery cross ring, and Morgan was wearing his cross necklace. All of his jewelry had been removed. This included his Garmin watch, which Dylan was keeping safe at home. Later, I would learn that some of the other items Bill had been wearing, like his running headband, were at home covered in blood, and Dylan had made sure to get those out of sight so that none of us would have to look at them.

At the hospital, there was a bag filled with more of his things. I opened it to see the running shirt inside. It had been cut off his body by the paramedics. I pulled out his running shoes and held them to my chest. I continued to beg God to let him live and be himself. That was the thing - I didn't just want him to live. I wanted him to be Bill, to have his mind, to be able to put on those shoes again.

All night, I took turns sitting on the cold recliner that didn't recline and standing next to Bill, holding his hand. When I sat on the recliner, I covered myself with those blankets that had covered him. I did not sleep.

Once upon a time, more than two decades before this, I remember being all worn out and exhausted from fighting cancer and taking care of him when he was sick and thinking, "I wish Bill were here to help me take care of this cancer patient." And here I was again, wishing Bill could be there to hug me and tell me I'm not alone.

But I was alone. I was all alone in a cardiovascular ICU on a cold chair, covering myself with blankets that had been on my dying husband, about to have the first of many sleepless nights ahead.

Just one night before, I was returning from a trip to Washington, D.C., where Bill and I had been lobbying for pediatric cancer. I was tired and so happy to be home, crawling into my bed. I was thinking about how I would spend Sunday preparing for the week ahead, and how I couldn't wait to pick up Bella, my mini schnauzer, who always slept in bed with Bill and me.

Morgan picked up Bella that night. I'm sure she was confused. She had been staying in the pet care facility where we take her when we travel. Now, she was being picked up and taken home, where neither Bill nor I was. And, instead of sleeping in our bed, she was sleeping in one of the upstairs guest rooms with Morgan. And the house was filled with people she loved, but we were nowhere to be found.

It was cold, dark, and scary in the ICU. The sounds of the many machines Bill was hooked up to became louder. There was constant commotion and beeping. Nurses and technicians were in and out all night long.

Finally, at 4:00 in the morning, following a sleepless and painful night, I walked out and asked someone if there was anywhere to get coffee, and they said that the cafeteria didn't open until 7:00. So I returned to sit on the cold, hard recliner where I was chilled to the bones and miserable.

I had no idea at the time how long this adventure would be and how much worse things would get at night in the ICU. Things would be much more frightening. I was facing profound fear and pain, and heading into the dark storm with no sleep and no coffee.

At 7:00, it was shift change. Bill was still unconscious and under the care of people who knew what they were doing. Why did I feel I needed to stay? I decided to go find coffee. There was a coffee stand in the main part of the hospital. I got a grande latte and returned to Bill's room, where I sat on the recliner and slowly warmed myself with my coffee. I also opened my laptop to see if I could get any work done.

The night before, I had an email sent to all of my authors letting them know that I would be moving slowly for a while but that the projects we were working on would get done, just not maybe when we had hoped to finish them. Bell Asteri Publishing and our advocacy were very important to us, and I was sad when I realized that this situation could mean having to turn it all over to someone else. It would be like giving away one of your babies!

Monday mornings are not anyone's favorite, but I looked out the window toward downtown Fort Worth and realized how extremely painful this one would be for Morgan. She had just moved to Fort Worth to start a new position at an oil and gas company downtown. We had all convinced her to go to work that day. There were many reasons for this. She had just been on the job for a week, and it would be very challenging to miss work when she had just started training. But more importantly, we all believed she needed to distract herself from her dad's condition and focus on working. I couldn't imagine how hard it was for her to get up and get dressed that morning and drive through traffic to work in a building just a block away from her dad's building. But she did it, and she didn't tell anyone there about the traumatic events of the past 24 hours, that her dad was maybe dying in a hospital ICU.

Dylan and my mom arrived that morning. Bill remained in a sedated and paralyzed state. This was purposeful as the cardiology team met to make decisions, and at the time, everything was based on brain function.

Jim and Eric from Bill's work asked for an update and to see if they could visit. I told them Bill was not conscious, but that absolutely, they could come to visit, and that it would likely be good for him. We needed anyone Bill knew well to come over to see if he could recognize them, to know his brain was functioning.

All day Monday, Bill was asleep, but there were glimpses that he was aware of us. There were little facial expressions, and I could just sense him in there, not dead. It was a long day. At some point, I forced myself to head home and grab our will. I needed to get my power of attorney out to let the hospital staff make a copy of it. Just opening the file was enough to make me want to vomit. This was not the first time I faced being a widow, but I wasn't feeling as strong now. Being 33 in the midst of a storm is different than being 55 in one. I felt my age.

I had begun texting friends to tell them what was happening. I couldn't even think about who all to tell. However, I realized that the news was getting out because I began receiving calls and texts. It was hard to decide not only who to tell, but if telling people was helpful or harmful. I didn't want to scare anyone, but I also didn't want to fight alone. Prayer is a powerful weapon in these moments. Some people think that saying, "My thoughts and prayers are with you," is meaningless. Maybe I agree about the thoughts part, but not the prayer part. I didn't need anyone sending "good vibes" or "thinking of you," but prayer works.

When you think about the entire situation, you can't help but realize that God is real. It's pretty hard to chalk it up to luck that two of the passersby the morning before, when Bill collapsed, were registered nurses who knew how to administer quality CPR. Luck didn't save him. Jesus did. Why does God choose to save some people and let others die? I don't know. It is not that He has more love for Bill than anyone else. But, for some reason, He chose to save Bill. At least, it kind of appeared that way. We couldn't be sure of the outcome, but so far, he was alive, and he seemed to recognize us.

On Tuesday, they began to wake him up. It was time to truly test that brain function, and that was the only thing that would give us hope. I saw his eyes open briefly, and I could tell he knew us. One of the physicians talked to him loudly and asked him to give a thumbs-up, and he did. Talk about excitement! I asked him to squeeze my hand over and over again, and nothing happened. Then I said, "Bill, if you can hear me, squeeze your right hand." That did the trick. He squeezed his right hand. My mom held her phone to his ear while my dad prayed for him.

Now that we knew he wasn't brain dead, that there was decent function, we were faced with a new enemy: staph infection in his lungs. There was no way they could open his chest and do major surgery on his heart while he had an infection. The infectious disease doctor came to talk to me and explained that they would be administering a strong antibiotic through his IV, and it would take seven days to rid him of the infection. This would mean an extended ICU stay and being on all those monitors for a long time as we waited for what they believed would be a triple bypass surgery.

Through all of this, I wished desperately that I could hear Bill's voice. I called his phone to hear his voicemail. It made me cry. I wished all of this to be a bad dream that I was about to wake up from. But the nightmare continued, and those nights in the ICU were about to get even more disturbing in ways I could never have imagined.

On Wednesday, they decided to try to remove Bill from the ventilator. I had no idea how traumatic that would be for him.

By this time, we knew he understood who we were and had enough brain function to feel scared and trapped. Extubation is no joke. He had been intubated since early Sunday morning. I had no idea whether he was in a lot of pain or cold or anything. I did know that his fever had spiked to over 103, so they had him wrapped in pads that were cold as ice. These pads monitored his temperature. When he cooled down, they heated up, and when his fever spiked, they cooled down. He was tied down to the bed, restrained in every possible way. This must have truly scared him. He looked scared.

The first attempt to remove the ventilator did not go well. He kept biting the tube. The nurse told me that to him, it felt like he was being choked to death. He wanted to swallow, but the tube would not permit it. His hands and feet were bound. He must have felt like he was in prison, being tortured (more on this later). Finally, we got him calmed down enough to remove the tube, and he was free.

He could not talk. But he could kind of whisper. He felt thirsty, but he wasn't permitted to drink anything. He was hungry because he hadn't eaten since Saturday, and that meal wasn't even a meal - just a few chips and guac. Bill was totally confused. But over time, that day, he began to whisper more. He knew us.

What all did he remember? Did he remember the heart attack? While he was dead, did he see a light at the end of the tunnel or have an out-of-body experience? Did he remember the times my mom played music in his ear when he was unconscious? Did he remember the visits from people?

Later that day, his voice got better and became a raspy type of voice like someone with a sore throat might have. He began to improve enough to have a visit from the physical therapist to help him into the recliner. Then, he saw a speech pathologist who tested his ability to swallow so that he could be permitted to drink water and eat. She began with ice chips, then moved to water, then to chocolate pudding, and when he passed all of those tests, she gave him a small bite of cracker. It was determined he could have a liquid diet.

But this was the beginning of a new kind of hell for me. Bill's memory was about five seconds long, and if we were lucky, it was a couple of minutes long. He would ask what happened, and we would tell him, and then we would have to tell him over and over again. Sometimes, he seemed to grasp it, and then other times, it seemed like he didn't comprehend the severity of his situation at all. One time, he asked how Dylan was doing in Pensacola. Our son is a naval aviator. I told him that Dylan had moved to Corpus Christi months ago and that he was in Fort Worth now because of the heart attack. Then he remembered Dylan was supposed to be flying a T6 in New Mexico, and I told him that wasn't happening because Dylan had to come to Fort Worth. He cried. He asked about Morgan's new job, somehow remembering that she had just begun at a Fort Worth company, and he cried, worrying that he was ruining her life and career.

There were many ups and downs. Visits from family and friends helped. But then there was the night. I left to go home one night to eat some dinner, and because I hadn't slept in so long, I had decided to stay home and sleep in my own bed. But as soon as I made that decision, I got a call from the ICU nurse telling me they needed me to come back and calm Bill down. He was freaking out, pulling out his tubes and catheter (ouch!), and saying he had been captured and was being held against his will.

Morgan and Dylan drove me to the hospital.

That was one of the worst nights in my entire life (and that is saying a lot because I have had some really bad nights in life). Bill was in a constant panic, completely confused. His memory was destroyed, and he truly believed he had been kidnapped and was being held against his will in a facility where evil experiments were being done on him. I kept trying to calm him down and said repeatedly, "Bill, it's me. I would never let any harm come your way. You had a heart attack, and this is a hospital. You will be having surgery to heal your heart. Morgan and Dylan and Linda, and all of us have been here, and we love you." It would work for a few minutes and then begin again.

Then he began to hallucinate. He saw dogs walking around everywhere. He thought we were in Florida on a beach and that a magic show with swords was happening. He saw a reindeer behind me trying to attack me. Sometimes, he would calm down and even fall asleep for a few minutes, and then wake up and try to get out of bed. That would make the alarms sound, and nurses would have to run and help me. Because he had yanked out his catheter, he was now having to pee in a urinal to measure his output. I tried to help him stay in bed to do this, but he would panic and try to get up. It was a constant battle. He would get up thinking that they had stolen his running clothes or Garmin or jewelry. I was in over my head. I didn't want them to restrain him, but if that was the only option, I would have it done. I did everything in my power to calm him all night long to avoid those restraints.

Pain. I have learned that physical pain is awful, but I have also learned that mental and emotional pain is even worse. I was now in pain in every possible way. Thursday morning, I desperately wanted some coffee, but once again, the cafeteria wasn't yet open, so I sat on the recliner, freezing and exhausted. And finally, at 7:00, I told the nurses, as their new shift was beginning, that I would be right back. I hoped that they could keep Bill calm long enough for me to pee and get some coffee.

Thursday was a mostly good day for Bill. It seemed like the day, with its natural light coming into the room, was good for him mentally. He had a lot of visitors on Thursday, including all of my siblings. It truly cheered him up. He and Dylan spent a lot of time together and had some great conversations. He was calm most of the day. It was good because he also had his first cognitive test with the speech pathologist, and he passed.

For three decades, Bill and I have had a tradition of writing each other a letter every Thursday. Our Thursday letters are very important to us. I could hardly keep up with what day we were on at this point, so I didn't expect Bill to remember. He couldn't remember what happened two minutes ago! What a sweet surprise when he asked Morgan and my sister, Anna, what day it was and said he needed to write me a Thursday letter.

Dylan told me to go home and sleep in my own bed that night. He promised to sit in that super uncomfortable recliner all night and take care of Bill. It was not easy for me to agree to this because I knew the nights were so scary, and I also hated that Dylan wasn't getting any sleep. Anna helped convince me to go.

It had been determined that Bill's bypass surgery would have to wait until Monday to give his lungs time to eliminate the infection. So, my mom drove back to Huntsville to take care of some things and even cook some meals for us. Anna, Morgan, and I went home, leaving Dylan with Bill. While Morgan went to spend a bit of time with a friend, my sister and I sat on the couch. She bought us dinner, and we watched *Modern Family* until finally, I went to bed.

It was nice to sleep in my bed with Bella, but I was filled with sorrow. Why on earth was this happening? We seem to get through one major traumatic event just in time for another. I won't stop having faith. Jesus said we would have trouble in this world. He was not kidding.

As I drifted off to sleep, I prayed for Dylan to be able to handle any challenges coming from Bill that night. Nights in the ICU with people dying and Bill panicking are not for the weak, and I am glad my son is brave and strong. And I was glad for a night away from it because I would need some strength for the coming days. And nights.

Preparing for Surgery

We needed Bill to get strong. We needed his brain to be functioning well, and for the infection in his lungs to clear so he could have bypass surgery.

On Friday morning, I arrived just before shift change and told Dylan to go home and sleep. I had slept for about five hours Thursday night, and that helped me feel so much stronger. This meant that I would be able to concentrate on helping Bill work on memory all day.

Dylan told me that although neither of them had slept a lot that night, Bill was more at peace. He had wanted to hear stories from Dylan about flying and some of the other pilots in the Navy. He was calmer and had an easier time accepting why he was in the hospital. His memory was still bad, but when Dylan explained what was happening, he believed him and didn't try to escape.

Someone suggested to Dylan that he create a timeline to help Bill remember things. This became a lifesaver over the next few days. Beginning with Saturday, March 1, Dylan wrote down the events of the days. Bill couldn't remember anything past

Wednesday, February 26. That was our first night in D.C. when we had dinner with our friends at District Taco. Bill couldn't remember anything else from that trip. He couldn't remember the many people we met and lobbied with. He couldn't remember the fun nights we had in the lobby of the hotel, talking to our Gold Together friends, or the trip home. He couldn't remember running with Morgan on Sunday, and he couldn't remember any of the visitors he'd had over the past few days. The timeline was a huge help, and in addition to writing down everything that had happened each day, we also recorded the names of all his visitors and those he talked to on the phone.

Later in the morning, Anna let her eight-year-old son, Cash, Facetime with Bill. Those tiny moments of cheer were good for him, strengthening him for open heart surgery. He was also being strengthened cognitively and able to pass higher-level tests. Sadly, I had to eventually ban him from using his phone and iPad because he was checking emails and sending messages that did not make sense. I also had to remind him repeatedly that he wasn't permitted to work.

His physical therapist came in twice that day to let him walk. He walked well. It felt like a huge victory and gave me hope that he would be fine. I still had the challenge of his memory, but this time, instead of having to tell him everything again, I would just hand him the timeline and let him read it. It reminded me of the movie *50 First Dates*. Bill was Drew Barrymore, and I was Adam Sandler, but none of this was funny. Well, some of it kind of was if I'm being honest.

I couldn't help but laugh when he constantly told people that he was going to be running a marathon the next month in Corpus, or that he had been at work all week and was now in

38

the hospital for a minor surgery. He was certain that he would have this "minor" surgery on Monday and that on Tuesday, he would be back at work. Then, I would have to tell him that he would not be back at work for several weeks. I would hand him the timeline and he would read it, look up at me shocked, and say, "I had a heart attack?" Then he would suggest that we ask for a second opinion.

It was strange that little moments of progress felt like big celebrations. When he was permitted to eat real food, we were so happy. He wished he could have coffee, but he wasn't permitted to have caffeine, and then they finally brought him some decaf coffee. What a huge smile he had! They were heavily monitoring his fluid intake, though, so we had to write down every amount of liquid that went in. We were also measuring everything that came out.

The hospital set up some educational videos for Bill and me to watch. Most of them were about the CABG (coronary artery bypass graft) and post-surgical care. It reminded me of two decades before, when we felt very lucky to be at MD Anderson Cancer Center, where we received an incredible education during cancer treatments. We love learning, and we have discovered that knowing what we are facing helps to lessen the fear.

Bill passed another cognitive test, this time a much higher-level test. I began to see his upbeat personality restored. I saw the guy who I saw decades ago - the one who never felt sorry for himself but did what he had to do to endure. As much as I hated all of this, I was glad to see him fight with joy.

Saturday, Bill had an ultrasound of his right arm. It was badly infected, and he was in a lot of pain. He had formed a blood clot from the IV, and it was decided that no more medication should go into that arm. He was pleading for some relief, but they told him that he was already on pain medication and the only thing they could do was wrap it with heat and ice alternately.

Bill was in great pain physically, but he was cheerful for the most part. He seemed to really be happy when people were there. The rules in the ICU were that only two people could visit at a time, but we broke those rules multiple times. The nurses didn't reprimand us. They seemed to like seeing Bill in that good mood, especially after those first few dreadful nights.

Bill, as always, loved getting to know the nurses and staff. We didn't get many breaks without the room being full of visitors and medical staff. I was so grateful to be in a place where it was obvious that he was receiving the absolute best care possible. I was also happy to know that Bill's heart surgeon, Dr. Macias, was listed as one of the top heart surgeons in the country. It made me feel safe.

Sunday was probably his most cheerful day. He was in agony physically because of his arm, but he had some great visits from family and friends. Virginia and Luke stopped by before they headed to the airport to go to Brazil. I know it was hard for them to leave the country when their brother-in-law was fighting for his life, but we promised to keep them updated.

Nurse Shay made my heart so happy that day, too. She decided to wheel Bill outside to the meditation garden. He hadn't been outdoors in so long, and he's an outdoor guy. It was not easy to get Bill out the door with all the machines he was hooked up to, but with two other nurses, Shay made it happen. Bill loved her. He convinced her to make her first visit to the Fort Worth Zoo, Bill's favorite zoo. He was having a happy day.

It was nice seeing him smiling, laughing, talking, and enjoying the day. You see, the next morning, he would have his chest sawed open, and I wanted him to be relaxed.

My mom returned that day. She, my kids, and I visited with him most of the day. Then they said their goodbyes while I stayed for a while longer. But I felt safe leaving him that night because he was at peace. His blood pressure was 114, and he was smiling. It had been a good day. He seemed to grasp the fact that he was facing surgery the next day, and he promised to behave that night. I kissed him and told him I would see him in the morning.

In bed that night, I struggled. I was scared. Suddenly, I felt overwhelmed. But I decided that my mind could destroy me, or I could choose to give it to God. I gave it to God and went to sleep.

An Open Heart

At 4:00 in the morning, I woke up. The darkness and fear I had felt the night before had calmed, but I was anxious. The night before, my mom, kids, and I had sat in the living room together. We had a quick prayer, and then we enjoyed some fun conversations about my mom and dad dating and falling in love. Dylan seemed to enjoy this conversation. Morgan seemed worried and didn't talk much.

We were all afraid of the unknown. Bypass surgery for anyone is scary, but Bill had already experienced sudden cardiac death. This was not a planned surgery. It was an emergency. I drank a cup of coffee in my bed and tried to pray, but all I could get out was, "God, please help."

When I arrived at the ICU, Bill was sad and in a great amount of pain. His blood pressure was very high, and he was the total opposite of the cheerful, peaceful guy I had left the night before. He finally had a nurse he did not like at all. She had ignored the orders to give him melatonin, and she had also neglected to see that she was not permitted to put anything into the IV line in his infected arm. She put magnesium into it, and it caused a shooting pain all up and down his arm. I had been kind and gracious to all the staff that whole week, but this was not ok. I called her in and asked why she had done this, and she acted like it was no big deal. But then I saw nurse Shay, who had cared for him the day before. It was about to be shift change, so I asked her to come in. I told her that I was upset because when I left Bill the night before, he was happy and calm and had low blood pressure, and now he was unhappy, had not slept all night, and was in great pain with high blood pressure. Shay was not happy to hear her orders for melatonin had been disobeyed, and she didn't know why the other nurse had put anything into that infected arm. This was not the way I wanted to start this very heavy day. I wanted him smiling and at peace like he was when I left. His life was on the line. They were about to saw open his chest bone and pull arteries from his legs. This was huge!

When the anesthesiology team came in, I had to sign many more papers. I had signed several the day before, consenting to the surgery. I had also given them my power of attorney. Now, I had to consent to anesthesia and sign that I understood the risk of death.

Dylan and I were there with him, and Bill enjoyed some light-hearted conversations with the anesthesiologist and nurses. I kissed his cheek. This time, instead of telling him to fight, I told him not to fight, to let Jesus fight for him. We wished him luck and told him we would see him in a few hours. As they wheeled him away, I wanted to run away somewhere and cry. I hadn't been able to cry too much, and I felt a desperate need to release it all. But I didn't. I watched him go down the hall and kept watching til he was out of sight. Just like I do when my kids come to visit, and when they leave, I watch til I cannot see their car any longer.

Dylan, my mom, and I sat in the waiting room for the next several hours. I thought about my words to Bill on the day his heart stopped beating: "Fight, Memo, fight!" And then I thought about my words to him that day: "Don't fight, Memo. Let Jesus fight for you."

THIS TIME, DON'T FIGHT!

When Bill had stage four cancer, it was a constant fight. One night, he had a dream that Jesus Himself showed up and handed him a sword, and that the two of them fought cancer cells together. I was thinking about how sometimes we face times when we need to fight. We need to be brave and strong and find the courage to face our enemy and fight to the finish. But there are other times when we need to lay down our weapons, be still, and let the Lord fight for us. And that was today. Bill needed to be still, to be at peace, to let a strong and powerful God fight the enemy.

Dylan and I were set up to receive text messages from the operating room with updates throughout the surgery. We had promised Morgan that every time we got a text, we would let her know. My mom brought us some quiche and sausage balls for us to snack on. I tried to relax and escape it all by watching *Modern Family,* and wouldn't you know.... one of the characters on the show was having heart problems! Why??????

As time went by, we got updates via text message from the operating room. For lunch, we used DoorDash and had Torchy's Tacos delivered. I wish I could say I felt peace, but I did not. I felt scared.

Finally, just over four hours later, Dr. Macias came to tell us that they had done four bypasses, not three. He said it all went well, that Bill would be on a ventilator for the next few hours, and that in about an hour, he would let us go see him. We felt relieved. Morgan arrived, and then she, Dylan, and my mom went to the meditation garden to walk around. I lay my head down on a chair to cry.

Soon, we were told we could go peek at him. All four of us walked back to his ICU room. He was still asleep, and he was hooked up to all kinds of monitors. Shay was with him. When a patient gets out of bypass surgery, the nurses have to sit with him and not leave. We could not walk into the room, just stand and look at him.

We went back and forth from the waiting room to the ICU room, but mostly, I stood outside his room watching him. I didn't want to leave him. And then he began to open his eyes. I talked to him and said, "Hi Bill." I asked, "Can you hear me?"

Bill slightly nodded, and then I asked if he could wave, and he did! I got Morgan and Dylan to come back to talk to him. We still couldn't enter the room, but we could stand right outside and talk. He began using sign language to communicate, just like we Gen Xers used to do in junior high school, across the classroom to each other.

Only a few hours after surgery, he was removed from the ventilator, and unlike the last time, this time, he could talk. His voice was raspy, but he could talk.

Soon, they let us go into the room and be next to him. Then Bill asked for something that was way out of character for him. He absolutely hates having his photo taken, but he asked the nurse if she would take a photo of all of us together. We were all smiles for that family shot.

I didn't want to leave, but he would be under constant care, so I kissed him goodbye and we left. What a relief. It was done.

Recovery

I imagine that everyone who undergoes open heart surgery has a lengthy recovery. In Bill's case, it was looking like that recovery period would be even longer than most because he'd had a heart attack with cardiac arrest.

On Tuesday morning, he was lucid, so I gave him back his phone. He would spend the next several days in the ICU before being transferred to a regular room on Thursday. And contrary to what they had predicted, he was discharged on Friday, one week ahead of their predicted schedule.

He was getting stronger. I saw my Bill, the one who wasn't afraid to get onto the back of a bull and ride, the one who decided to become an Ironman after three years of chemotherapy, the one who always refuses to let the troubles of life own him. Determination. That's Bill.

The day before being discharged, on Thursday, March 13, Bill, Morgan, Dylan and I sat in his hospital room and ate dinner together. We had some light, easy conversation and did some laughing. We told Bill about the weird parking garage at the hospital, where you never knew if you would have to pay or not or if so, how much. And how you could remember where you parked because each floor was named after an animal. Dylan said he didn't like parking on the Longhorn level and felt tempted to saw off those horns (only Aggies will understand this).

Morgan and Dylan also told Bill how they had gone running along the Trinity River with a running club the night before. We all agreed that we would get back. It wasn't over just yet.

On Friday morning, I dropped Dylan off at the airport and then went to the hospital to wait for Bill to be discharged. The nurse came in to remove the bandage on his chest. I was really amazed that it looked so clean. It was big, but it wasn't as ugly as I thought it would be. After lunch, he was allowed to dress in normal clothes, and then he was released.

We made it home, where our dog Bella wanted to jump on him immediately. I told her to be super calm while we got him on the couch. Then I put her into his lap. She wanted to lick his wounds - his chest and the wounds on his stomach and legs. If she could have gotten to the back of his head, she would have probably tried to get those stitches out too. She seemed to sense that he'd been hurt and she wanted to fix him.

Bill slept on the couch for a while and then decided to get up and take his first shower since March 1.

I created some charts to help me give him his many medications and monitor his weight and blood pressure. I went to grab his prescriptions and buy a new blood pressure monitor as ours had broken. Walgreens had messed up the prescriptions, thinking they could fill them days later, but thankfully, I had his discharge papers with me to prove he was supposed to be taking them immediately. So, I had to wait an hour with Bill at home alone. During that wait, I saw a line of people waiting to get prescriptions, and I started wondering what all they were for. I also began to feel the heaviness of the last two weeks sitting on my chest like an elephant.

The next several days consisted of not much sleep, pain, lots of medications, and a few easy walks around the block. No one had prescribed pain medication for Bill, but I called our friend Roger, a physician in Houston, to ask if Tylenol was appropriate, and he said it was.

I finally felt comfortable leaving Bill for short periods to run errands, and I even went to the gym to swim laps with Morgan. It was not easy to leave him, but I made sure he had his phone, and I knew our neighbors would be there in a second if anything happened.

Sometimes, I think I missed my calling in life and that I should have been a physician or nurse. I've learned a lot about caregiving. And I certainly have kept my vows about loving my husband in sickness and in health. I spent the next several days administering his medications, getting him to follow-up appointments, walking with him, planting the garden with him, and listening to music on the couch. We learned a lot about moving slowly. He was not permitted to work or even think about work - doctor's orders! So, we learned a lesson about being slow and relaxing, about forgetting the world for a minute and hitting the "refresh" button. Home. It had a different feel all of a sudden.

Good Samaritans

I had kept the phone number of Miranda, one of the nurses who had administered CPR on Bill. I also found the other nurse, Karen, and the young family who stopped to help that day through our neighborhood HOA Facebook page. I reached out to them all to thank them and update them on Bill.

On Sunday, March 23, exactly three weeks after he died on the street, Bill asked me to take him back to the spot where it all happened. He stood there in awe. There was a tiny bit of his blood still on the sidewalk. We both realized that this place would never be the same to us again. In fact, we will never be the same again. How could we?

I remembered how, a couple of weeks before, Morgan was driving me along that street and got very suddenly angry and panicked and pulled over. She jumped out of her SUV, and I followed her. We stood on this exact spot, and I told her we were reclaiming this little place on the sidewalk. I said, "We won't look at this as the place where your daddy died. Instead, this is the place where your daddy's life was saved! God showed up right here, and when Death came to take him, Jesus breathed life into him. It is a special place, a good place, a place to cherish."

You know, that was easy to say, but I had to decide to believe my own words. There are pictures you can't get out of your head ever. My daughter will never forget what she witnessed there on March 2, 2025. She watched her dad fall down and die. I won't ever forget it either. I was picked up by a woman I didn't know and drove up to a scene with flashing lights and paramedics on top of my husband, who was lying on the ground.

But I will do my best to remember that in our darkest moment, Jesus Himself showed up. He was on that sidewalk. He heard us cry out, and He answered our cry.

I cannot begin to imagine what it felt like for Bill to stand there. He has no memory of that day. But it's a place he won't look at the same either. While he stood there, he thanked God for saving him and asked Him to help him know his purpose for being here.

We left that day to head to Miranda's house. She lived around the corner from us, and it was incredible introducing Bill to one of the women who saved his life. She and her husband were both home, and they both are registered nurses at a trauma center. We sat on their couch and chatted for a while. Miranda told us that on the morning of March 2, she normally didn't drive that way, but that she had decided to head that way to go to Home Depot before church. She just happened to drive by at the exact time when she was needed. She is one of my heroes.

I think the word "hero" gets misused, or at least overused. We call athletes and movie stars heroes. There is nothing heroic about them. They may be idols, but heroes? No. Miranda is a hero. She literally saved my husband's life. Had she shown up just one minute later, he might not have made it. Her CPR, along with Karen's, was the reason oxygen went to his brain when his heart wasn't beating and he couldn't breathe on his own. Karen didn't normally go that way on Sunday mornings either, but just happened to drive by moments after Bill fell to the ground, and she decided to start CPR right away. The Thomison Family, including Jackie III, Misty, Jackie IV, and Scarlett, was heading to church and drove by as Bill collapsed. They didn't let Morgan fight alone. They prayed for her and comforted her through one of the most devastating moments of her life. Bill got to meet all of these heroes!

Thank you, Miranda. Thank you, Karen. Thank you, Jackie and Misty, and your precious little children, Jackie and Scarlett. Thank you to the paramedics. Thank you to Dr. Macias, Dr. Amin, and all of the physicians on the cardiology team. Thank you to nurses Shay and Katie and Mallory and Casey, and all of the incredible nurses and technicians, and staff at Texas Health Harris Methodist Hospital. You saved a life.

And thank you to our friends, family, and neighbors for the prayers and gifts, and for the constant love and support.

I do not know what is coming next. Recovery from sudden cardiac death, followed by quadruple bypass surgery, is not easy, but life is not easy. Life is hard. God spared my husband once again when Death tried to take him and the grave tried to swallow him up. There must be a reason, and we will know it soon.

THE BEAT GOES ON...

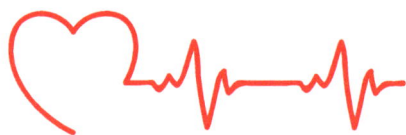

Photos

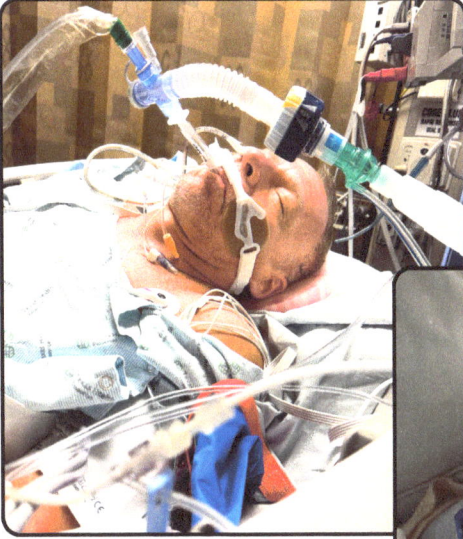

Sunday, March 2, 2025 in the
cardiovascular ICU

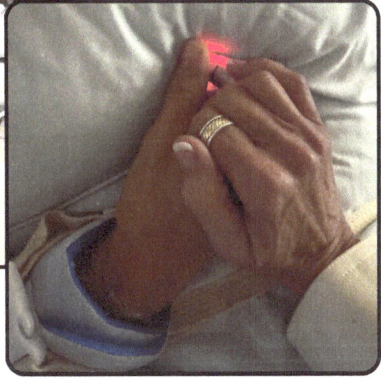

Holding Bill's hand while wearing
his wedding band

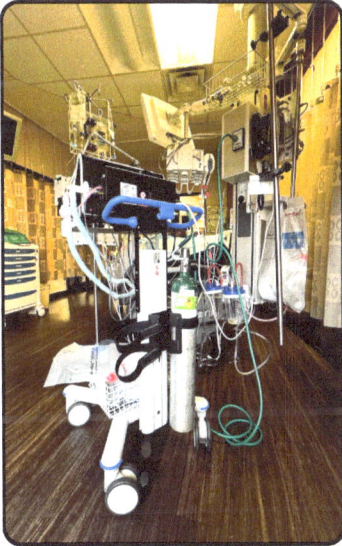

So many machines
keeping him alive

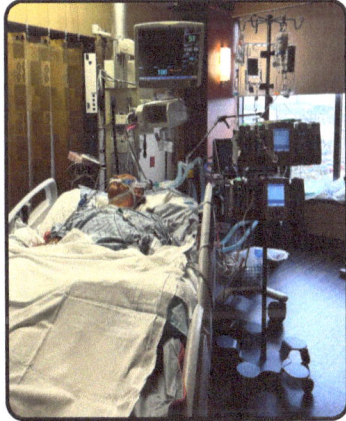

Fight, Memo, Fight!

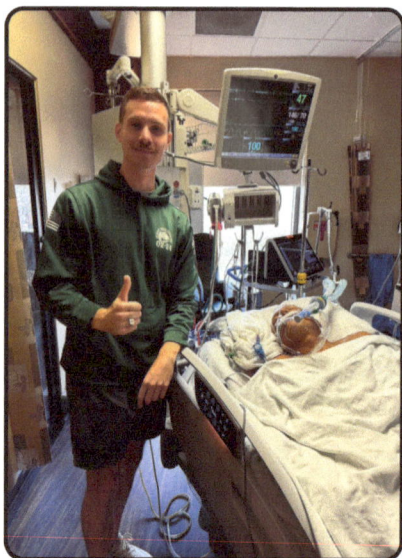
Dylan visiting his dad

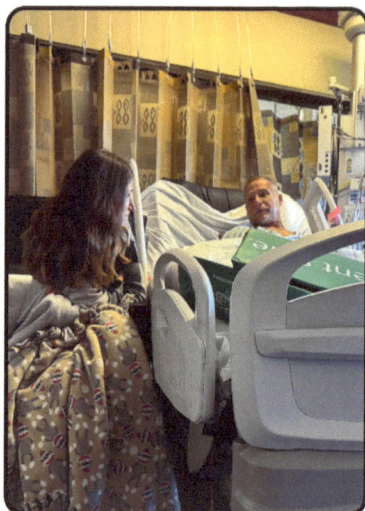
Morgan visiting her dad

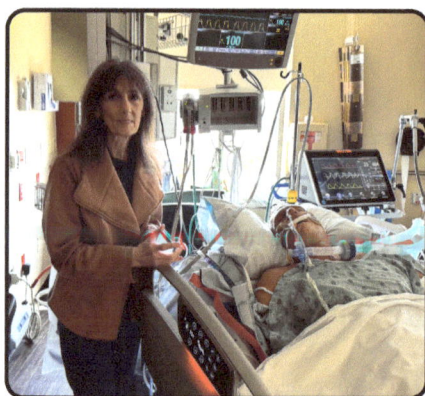
Linda visiting her son-in-law

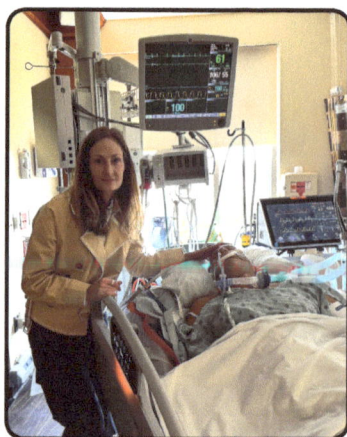
DS visiting her husband

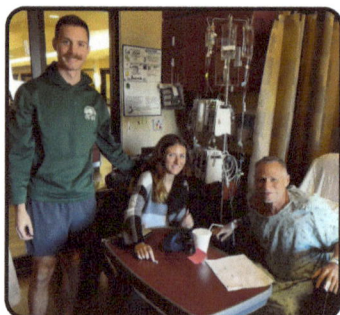
Bill feeling upbeat because
his kids are with him

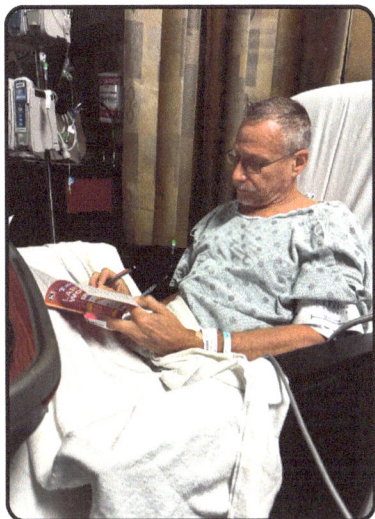

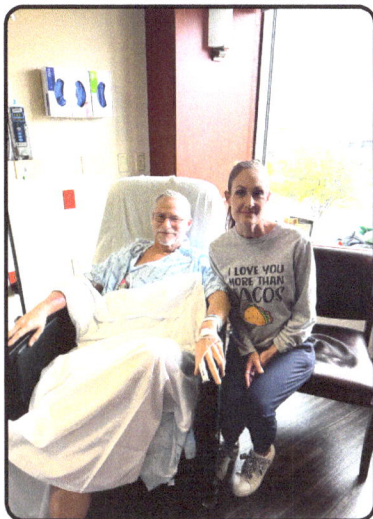

Finally getting to sit in the recliner and not be in the bed for a while

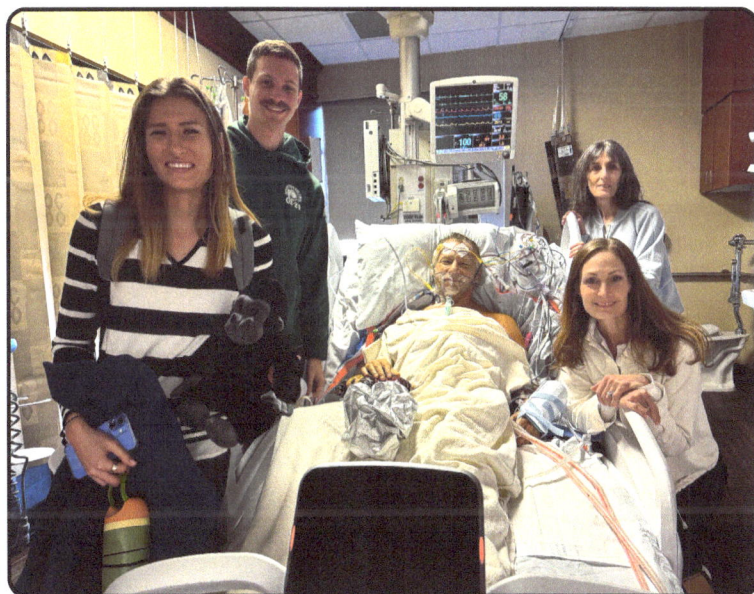

A few hours after bypass surgery and a request for a family photo

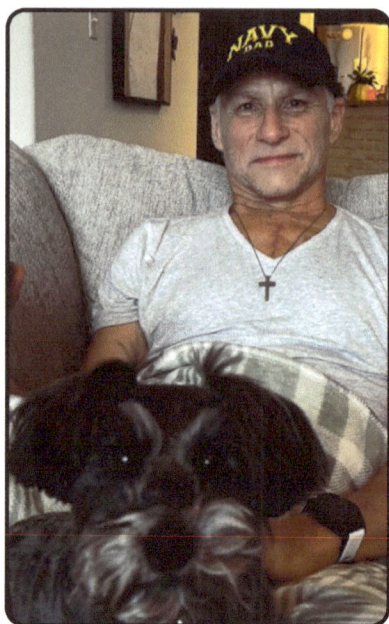

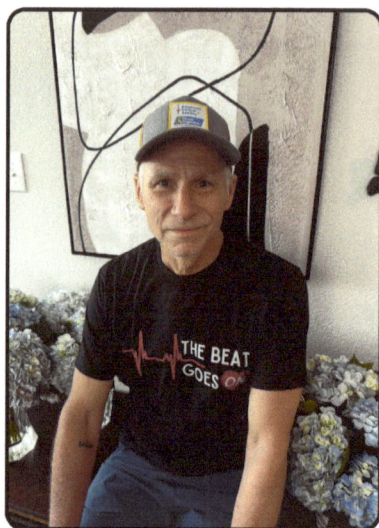

Following his first one-mile walk!

Home!

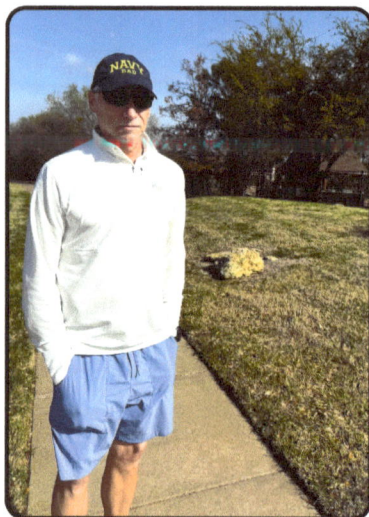

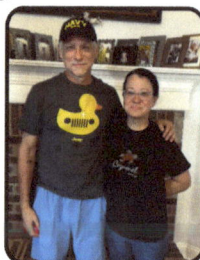

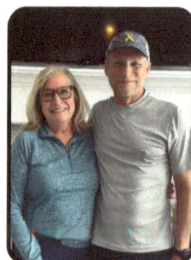

Meeting Miranda

Meeting Karen

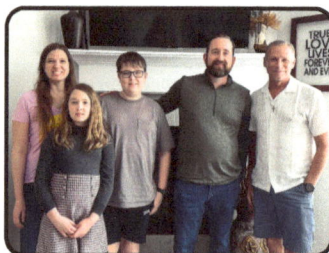

Returning to the spot where he
died three weeks before

Meeting the Thomison Family
(Misty, Scarlett, Jackie, and Jackie)

**The LORD will fight for you;
you need only to be still**

Exodus 14:14

contact the author at
dcrews@bellasteri.com

For more information about other books, visit...

www.ashlandink.com

or

www.bellasteri.com